Survival Medicine:

Useful Medical Handbook For Your Survival Medicine Kit

Disclamer: All photos used in this book, including the cover photo were made available under a Attribution-NonCommercial-ShareAlike 2.0 Generic and sourced from Flickr

Table of Contents

Survival Medicine: 1
    Useful Medical Handbook For Your Survival Medicine Kit 1
Introduction 3
Chapter 1 - Major Areas of First Aid in Case of Disaster 5
Chapter 2 - Important Medicines for First Aid Kit 12
Chapter 3 - Essential Things for the Treatment of Injuries 16
Chapter 4 - Medications for CPR and Stroke Treatment 18
Chapter 5 - Treatment for Poisons, Stings, and Bites, Freezing 24
Conclusion 34

Introduction

A well-stocked survival medicine kit is an important part of your life because it proves helpful in emergency situations. A properly designed first aid kit can help you to save the life of your family members.

A first aid kit contains all supplies in one location and you can easily access it to save an injured person. A good survival medicine kit will help you to save money and time. A ready-made first aid kit is available in the market, but it will be beneficial to prepare your own kit.

It will enable you to keep customized items in your first aid kit, such as medical suture, bandages, antiseptic, arm splints, pain medication, prescription medication, emergency tourniquet, burn salve, tweezers, etc.

There are some first aid treatments and techniques that you should learn to manage different wounds and health problems immediately. It is important to learn dressing, treatment for fever, burns, injuries and poisoning.

In an emergency situation, it is essential to learn different techniques to handle the situation. There are a few skills that you should learn to treat minor injuries and deep wounds to stop bleeding.

With the help of this survival medicine kit, you can treat traumas because untreated trauma can be horrifying. You can use different tools and medications of your survival medicine kit to increase chances of survival.

This book is meant to share important details about survival medicine kit. This medical handbook is good for your guidance to design your own first-aid kit. After reading this book, you will be able to help your friends and family members in a survival situation.

Chapter 1 – Major Areas of First Aid in Case of Disaster

There are a few tips that will help you to treat major areas in case of disaster to protect your family:

Short Breathing

A runny nose, nasal congestion, itchy eyes, cough, chest congestion, labored breathing, shallow breathing and wheezing are some common symptoms of short breathing. Some toddlers may experience occasional breathing problems. These are caused by viral infection, cold, viral bronchitis, etc. Some other conditions are seasonal allergies, asthma, and pneumonia.

Steps to Treat Short Breathing

There are some simple steps that will help you to treat short breathing problems in toddlers, such as:

- Offers extra fluid, such as water and juice to your patient. It will loosen mucus and avoid any infection linked to dehydration. The fluid will not defeat the virus, but it can reduce the discomfort and avoid complications.

- A cool-mist humidifier is necessary for the room of your toddler. It can moist the air and increase the comfort of a sick patient. It is useful to treat respiratory illness, such as seasonal allergies.

- It will be good to give a ½ teaspoon of honey to your toddler for a cough and chest clogging. It is a safe home remedy for the patient, but it may not be good for infants younger than 12 months.

- The home physical therapy will help you to loosen phlegm from the chest of your toddler. Let your patient lay down (face-down) and tap his/her back with a cupped hand. It will help toddlers to expel and remove thick mucus in the trachea and lungs.

- You should talk to the licensed pediatrician of your toddler before using herbal supplements for the treatment of respiratory diseases.

Choking

The symptoms of choking are:

- Your patient is unconscious
- Unable to breathe properly because the airway is blocked
- Wheezing and gasping
- Unable to cry or talk
- Face turning blue
- Grabbing at the particular area of throat

Call for emergency and during this period, you should start CPR:

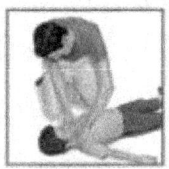 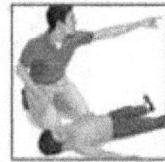
Tap and shout

Yell for help. Send someone to phone 911 and get an AED

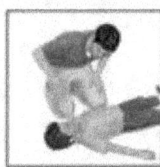 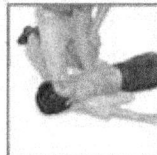
Look for no breathing or only gasping

Push hard and fast. Give 30 compressions

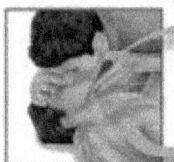 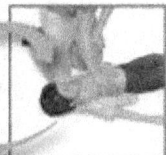
Open the airway and give 2 breaths

Repeat sets of 30 compressions and 2 breaths

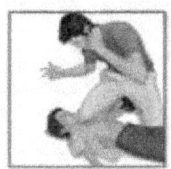 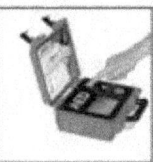
If you are alone after 5 sets of 30 compressions and 2 breaths, phone 911, and then resume sets of 30:2

When the AED arrives, turn it ON and follow the prompts

Set Your Patient into Position

Hold your patient while keeping his/her face down with your arms and support with thigh:

Keep the torso higher than the head

Forceful Blows

You will use the heel of your hand to thump the patient between the shoulders for almost five times.

Turn the patient's faces up while giving support to the neck and head. If the object is not out, move to another step.

Press the Chest

Keep your patient on a flat surface and put your three fingers in the center of the breastbone of your patient and quickly push for almost five times.

Replicate the back thumping and pushes on the chest, until the object is out and the patient loses consciousness.

If the patient is unable to breathe, open the airway with the help of your thumb. Put your thumb in the mouth and grasp e lower gums or incisors. The jaws should lift up to look for the object.

It is not good to pull the object out because it can accidentally push the object deeper into the throat of the patient.

Nosebleed

For the treatment of nosebleed, let your patient sit upright, but don't tilt her head to the back. Remove or loosen any tight band or cloth around the neck.

Pinch the lower part of the nose nearby nostrils and let him/her lean forward while applying pressure for 5 to 10 minutes. You shouldn't release it because it can prolong the bleeding. Make sure to get medical help immediately to avoid any major problem.

If the nosebleed is due to a trauma, you can use an ice pack to reduce swelling. Once the bleeding is slow down, keep the ice pack against the bridge of the nose. If the situation persists after ten minutes, call your doctor to check for an internal injury.

First Aid for Broken Bones

Patient under the age of five years have chances of injuries and accidents at home. The Younger patient is unable to assess dangers because of lack of development and experience.

Injuries occurred in the home are linked to the age of the patient and the level of development. In the early ages, the babies are able to grasp, wriggle and chew. The patient may suffer from different bone fractures and injuries. There are some steps that will help you:

Symptoms

- A snap of grinding noise during the injury
- Swelling, tenderness and bruising
- Difficult to move a particular part of the body
- Can't bear weight and touch

What to do?

- Carefully remove the clothes from the injured area and apply an ice pack wrapped in the cloth
- Place the injured limb in its position as you find it. Keep a simple splint on the broken area because the splint will keep the bone still and protect it until you get medical help.
- Make sure to prevent any movement of the injured part because it can cause serious damage. Immediately call emergency (911) or others in your area.
- If the patient has an open break, such as the bone is obtruded through the skin with bleeding, apply pressure to the bleeding area with a clean piece of cloth or other material. There is no need to wash the wound or put back the part of the bone.

Temporary Splint

You can use a small cardboard, board or newspaper to wrap it with an elastic band or tape.

Note: Keep your patient lying down until you get medical help. If your patient has a lightheaded feeling, you can keep the head at a lower level than the chest. It will be good to lift the legs, if possible.

It will be good to keep the injured part above the level of the heart to relieve swelling. You should avoid heat for at least 24 hours after injury because it can increase pain and swelling. The use of ibuprofen will be good to relieve pain.

Chapter 2 – Important Medicines for First Aid Kit

There are a few things that should be there in your survival medicine kit to stop bleeding protect wounds and avoid infections.

Duct Tape

You should keep a duct tape because it is a life saver and help you to deal with cut and wounds. It can be quickly pulled out to cover an open wound to stop bleeding and avoid infection.

Butterfly Sutures

These are great to close up small wounds because these adhesive strips can be used together to cover a wound. Before using it or duct tape, you should carefully clean your wound and wash out debris.

If you have any kind of antiseptic, you should apply it on the wound and let the area dry. You can bring two sides together and tape them to shut.

Tips to Avoid Infection

A survival situation will increase lots of sanitation issues and you should keep your wounds clean and covered. It is extremely important because the infection can be triggered on the top of open wounds. You should carry the following items with you:

- Adhesive dressings for wounds

- Gauze

- Antibiotic creams and ointments

- Oral antibiotics, such as Ciprofloxacin, Erythromycin, and Amoxicillin

- You will need disinfectants and antiseptics, such as PVP iodine Ampules, Peroxide, Isopropyl and Antiseptic wipes.

Items for the Management of Pain

You should keep items for the management of pain because sometimes, the pain can be deadly and unbearable. It is important to keep medicines to manage pain and decrease inflammation. Your emergency survival kit should include:

- Codeine or another painkiller

- Aspirin, Ibuprofen or Tylenol

- Ice Bags

- Lidocaine

Important Things to Deal with Allergies

There are certain kinds of things that can be the reason of allergies and you should keep medicines to fight with allergic reactions. If you don't have certain kinds of allergies, still you should keep medicines for allergies in your survival kit.

If you have food allergies, these can cause anaphylaxis reactions that should be treated immediately. Your kit should have:

- Antihistamine or Benadryl aka Diphenhydramine HCl should be in your kit.
- Creams for Antihistamine
- EpiPen aka Epinephrine is essential to treat severe allergy. It is good to control the anaphylaxis reaction.

Specific Items for Unique Medical Needs

You should give special attention to your health and for this purpose; there are a few medications for your kit:

- You should keep the extra prescribed medication in your stock to treat different medical conditions.
- OTC medications are also required to treat nausea, arthritis, etc.

Essential Items for Kit

Your survival medicine kit should contain following items:

- Emergency dental kit
- Surgical blades
- Sterile needles
- Quick Clot Gauze
- Splints – SAM
- Grooming Tools

- Cleaning tools, such as nail clippers, bath soap, and Antiseptic wipes.
- Scissors
- Tweezers
- Disposable gloves
- Disposable thermometers
- Sterile eyewash
- Eye dressings
- Vaseline
- Sun block
- Burn creams along with dressings
- Medical manuals with basic first aid instructions

You should keep all these items in your first aid kit for treatment of different health problems and injuries.

Chapter 3 – Essential Things for the Treatment of Injuries

In a survival situation, you may get different injuries and wounds. There are a few essential tools that should be an important part of your medicine kit:

Tweezers

You should keep them in your first aid kit while enjoying hiking and other outdoor activities. This is a secure way to remove ticks and splinter with a pair of tweezers. Make sure to disinfect your tweezers well before and after every use.

Hydrocortisone Cream

If you want to treat itchy bites, you can keep two packets of this cream. This topical steroid treatment helps you to get quick relief from itching and get rid of the inflammation.

Glove and Hand Sanitizers

If you or your friend gets a wound, you should not touch it with dirty hands. You should clean your hands with a sanitizer in the absence of soap and water. You should keep a pair of non-latex and latex gloves. Wear gloves, sanitize your hands and now treat any wound.

Pain Relievers

A first aid kit is incomplete without these medications, such as acetaminophen, aspirin, and ibuprofen. These are good to treat fever and pain. You should keep these medications in your first aid kit. The aspirin is not good for a person under 18 years of age because it can cause Reye's syndrome.

Tape and Gauze

Scrapes and cuts should be treated with gauze pads and taps because these will help you to stop bleeding from a small wound. These can be used as bandages to protect scraps, cuts, and wounds.

Wipes and Solutions to Clean Wounds

You should clean your wounds and scrapes with the help of wipes and solutions to protect it from germs and infections. It is essential to keep antiseptic sprays for hand injuries. Saline solutions and sterile water are also required to wash your eyes injuries and wounds.

Antibiotic Cream

You should keep an antibiotic cream or ointment because it has several uses. It can protect wounds from infection and keep the particular area moisturized. In its presence, your wound will not be attached to a bandage.

Chapter 4 – Medications for CPR and Stroke Treatment

If you want to treat a patient suffering from stroke, you can follow the given instructions:

Treatment for Heat Stroke

Heat stroke aka hyperthermia is a condition in which the body temperature dramatically increases to its highest level. It should be treated properly; otherwise, it could be fatal. The dramatic increase in body temperature may be due to dehydration.

Symptoms

- Disorientation
- Confusion
- Absence of sweating
- Agitation
- Coma
- Headache
- Fainting
- Weakness
- Increased thirst
- Vomiting and nausea

- The temperature will be 105°F (40.5°C) or higher
- Flushed and dry skin
- Seizures
- Loss of consciousness
- Rapid breathing and rapid heartbeat

What to do?

If you notice any of these symptoms in your patient, you should seek emergency help. There are some treatments that you can do while awaiting medical help for your patient:

- Bring your patient in the shade without wasting time
- Remove dress of your patient
- Make your patient lie down and keep feet slightly elevated
- If the patient is alert, you can keep it in the cool water. If you are away from your house, make sure to spray water on your patient with a hose.
- If possible, let your patient frequently sip clear and cool fluids
- In the case of vomiting, turn the side of your patient to avoid choking.

Prevention for Heatstroke

- If you want to avoid heatstroke, let your patient drink plenty of water during hot and sunny weather, even without feeling thirsty.
- Make sure to select light-colored and loose clothes for your patient in hot weather.
- Make sure to prevent your patient from participating in any heavy outdoor activity during the hottest hours of the day.
- Teach your patient to immediately come indoors when they feel overheated.

CPR Treatment

Any blockage in the supply of blood is a big reason for a heart attack. There are serious risks, such as the heart may stop beating and it is known as cardiac arrest. If you notice these symptoms in a person, he/she is getting a heart attack:

- Continuous pain in chest and it may spread to the jaw, arms, and neck.
- Pale skin
- Weak and rapid pulse
- Sweating and perspiration

If you are noticing these symptoms, you should give CPR treatment to patient, such as:

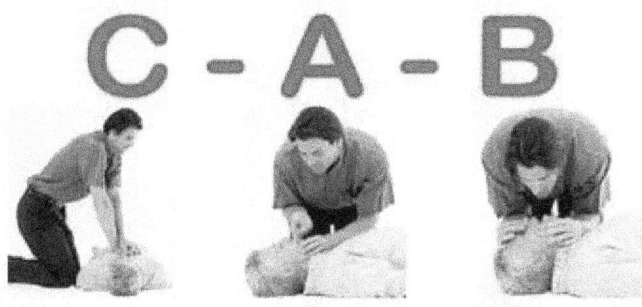

Shock

If you want to give shock, follow the given instructions:

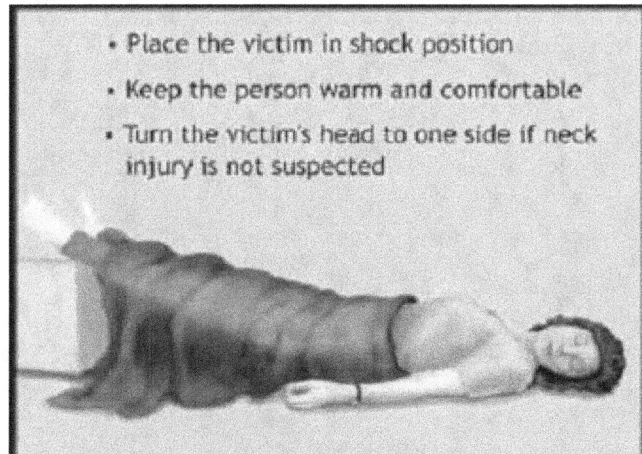

You should follow these steps that will help you to give instant first aid to patients suffering from first aid.

High Fever

Fever is a high temperature in which the body temperature goes above the 37°C (98. 6°F). It is caused by a sore throat, infection, chickenpox, and earache. It is common in children and should be treated immediately because the temperature above 39°C (102.2 °F) can be dangerous for a child.

Symptoms

There are six important things to look if someone has a fever:

- High temperature more than 37°C (98. 6°F)
- Cold with shivering body and chattering teeth
- Pale skin
- Sweating, hot and flushed skin
- General aches
- A headache and pain

Who to do?

If you notice your child suffering from fever, you should help them to stay comfortable. Give them water to avoid any problem from the loss of moisture via sweating. You can give them recommended a dose of paracetamol but avoid aspirin.

Check pulse, breathing and response of the patient

You can use antibiotic for a bacterial infection. It will be good to use ibuprofen, but avoid aspirin for teens and children.

Chapter 5 – Treatment for Poisons, Stings, and Bites, Freezing

Poisoning may cause you death due to inhaling, swallowing, and injection, touching and inhaling various venoms, chemicals, drugs, and gasses. There are a few cleansers that are dangerous to ingest and these should be kept away from your children.

First Aid for Poisoning

Almost 90 percent of the childhood poisonings happen at home and it should be treated according to the advice of poison control center.

The sudden changes in the behavior of your child, drowsiness, excessive drooling, confused mental state, vomiting, fragments of pills on clothes and lips, confused mental state, lethargy, etc. These all are symptoms of poisoning.

What to do?

If you suspect that your child has taken a poison, you should contact your local poison control center. It is important to remember specific container or bottle of the substance ingested by your child.

Prevention:

- It is important to keep medicines locked in cabinets.
- Keep cleaning products and alcohol away from the reach of your children.
- Discard used batteries and buttons to keep them far from your children.
- It is not good to tempt your child by telling that the medicine tastes like a candy.
- The poison should not be kept on the floor.

Tips to Do while Waiting for Help

If you are waiting for help for a person swallowed poison, you can perform the given activities:

If the person has swallowed poison, remove any remaining thing in the mount of this person. If the person has swallowed household cleaner or chemical, carefully read the label and follow the instructions given for any accident of accidental poisoning.

Remove any remaining poison on the skin after wearing gloves. Rinse the skin with water for 15 to 20 minutes under a hose.

If the poison is in the eye, carefully flush the eye with lukewarm or cool water for 20 minutes or until you gets help.

In the case of poison inhalation, you should take affected person in the fresh air and if the person vomits, turn his/her head to the side to avoid any choking.

Treat Insect Bites and Stings

If your patient has been stung or bitten, you can notice swelling on face, dizziness, fainting or difficult breathing. There could be a serious allergic reaction along with extreme pain and irritation. You should call a doctor if the patient is bitten near the mouth.

What to Do:

Remove the stinger on the skin and slightly scrape the area with a credit card or fingernail. It is not good to pinch the stinger with tweezers of your fingers. It can spread venom in the body.

Clean the Area

- Use mild soap and water to clean the area and treat the symptoms.
- In the case of itching, use a cold compress on the area for almost one minute and use calamine lotion or a cream (1% hydrocortisone). It shouldn't be used on a broken skin.
- Remove any tight jewelry from the bitten area, but be careful because it will be difficult to remove due to swelling.
- Use ice in the particular area for 10 minutes and then removes the ice for 10 minutes. Repeat this procedure for several times.
- If the area is elevated, it means the sting is in this area.

- You can use ibuprofen or acetaminophen for the patient to relieve pain. It is important to follow instructions given on the bottle or call your pediatrician.
- It will be good to use a mixture of water and baking soda or calamine lotion for itching.

How to apply ice without irritating your patient?

Sometimes, the patients are not able to bear ice pack. You can use a thin plastic bag or a dry washcloth to wrap the ice. The use of animal-shaped compresses can make your work easy because patient likes to use these things.

It will be good to use books, small toys, bubbles or colorful stickers to distract your small patient. The patient between 6 to 12 years of age can be distracted via portable games, music, stories and TV shows.

Frostnip: It is the mildest freezing cold wound and the ear lobes, cheeks, noses, fingers and toes are its main victims. These parts of the body become more exposed to the cold. The color of affected area may turn white and numb. The top layer of the skin becomes hard and the deeper tissues become soft.

You can prevent this problem by using warm clothes and shoes. Gentle rewarming may help you to treat the affected skin. It is a cold-induced injury, and the affected part should not be rubbed because the ice crystal can damage the skin. The use of the very hot warm bottle is not also good for the treatment of frostnip.

Frostbite: It is a common injury as a result of extreme cold and objects made of metal. It can be caused by the normal temperature from the contact with compressed gasses. The temperature below freezing point 0°C/32°F can be the reason for this problem because it can obstruct the blood flow.

It may result in the severe and permanent damage to the blood circulation. In several cases, the permanent damage and restriction in the blood circulation may occur. The inflammation of the skin is the symptom of mild infection that may accompany with slight pain. In various cases, the tissues may damage with prickling sensation. This may also cause blisters. The frostbitten skin may prone to get infection and death of soft and local tissues and hindrance in blood supply.

First Aid for Frostbite

If a part of your skin turns white and hard, then these can be the symptoms of frostbite. In order to treat frostbite, you may follow the following first aid tips:

Seek permanent medical care by going to a doctor or a hospital. If it is not possible to see the doctor immediately, then you can try the followings:

Restore Warmth

- Arrange a warm place for the patient and remove wet clothing if any.
- The person should avoid walking on the frostbitten toes or feet.
- Try to arrange proper warmth for the patient, and don't reward until you have a proper solution to keep it constantly warm. Keep it in mind that the warming and then the re-exposure in the cold temperature of the frostbitten area may cause worse damage.

- Use warm water to keep the area gently warm and continue this treatment until the skin becomes red and warm.
- If you found no water close to, you can breathe the area by cupping it with your hands and hold it next to the body.
- Direct heating pads and radiators are not good to use.
- Avoid massage otherwise your skin may get blisters.

Bandage the Area

- Use dry and sterile dressing and apply it loosely.
- Try to keep the fingers and toes separate by keeping clean cotton balls between them.
- It is good to get access to the hospital as soon as possible because the doctor will provide better treatment like rewarm the area, tetanus vaccine or any other medication.

First Aid for Hypothermia

Hypothermia is a condition of the body when it loses heat at a faster rate as compared to its production rate. The exposure to cold weather is the basic reason behind it. Shivering, temperature drops, slurred speech, shallow breathing, weak pulse, loss of consciousness and red skin are its common symptoms.

Seek Emergency Medical Care

If you find a patient suffering from hypothermia, call 911 or the local emergency number, and take the following steps on an immediate basis:

Try to find a warm corner and move the person from the cold. It is important to protect a person from the wind and cover the neck and head area. Provide insulation on the cold ground.

Find out if there are warm and wet clothes, try to remove them and apply the dry compresses on the body. You can also use an electric blanket, hot water bottle or hot chemical packet.

You can provide a warm, but a non-alcoholic drink for the person. You can give CPR treatment to the person if you find no signs of life.

Follow Several Cautions

- You need to be careful because you can't rewarm the person quickly with a hot bath.
- Heating or massaging on the limbs of a person may increase the stress on the heart.
- Alcohol and cigarettes should be avoided because these can make the situation worst.

Treatment for Gas Inhalation

Inhalation of gas, such as carbon monoxide can be fatal for anyone because it can dramatically reduce the oxygen in your body. You should take the patient in the open air to get fresh air.

Burning padding, plastic material, and wood may create dangerous smoke. You should avoid this smoke and if you inhale these gasses accidently, there are a few treatments for you:

- Suspect requires immediate medical attention, so call a doctor
- Check the body of victim for any burns
- Transfer the victim to a safe place to get some fresh air
- Check for burns and injuries
- Stay with your victim until you get professional help

Nonfreezing Cold Injuries

Following are some nonfreezing cold injuries, and you should know about them:

Chilblains: These are mild cold injuries may be caused by the prolonged exposure to the cold for several hours. The air temperature may go above the freezing point and cause swelling, tingling and pain in the affected skin areas.

Immersion foot: It happens to the people with wet feet for days or a week with the temperature up to 10°C (50°F). It can basically injure nerve and muscle tissues. The itching, swelling, pain, and tingling is some symptoms of immersion foot. Initially, the skin may turn red or blue because of the injury progress.

Trenchfoot: It is a wet cold disease caused due to the extended exposure to the damp environment from above the 10°C (50°F). Its symptoms may appear in several hours, and take almost three days to recover. You can prevent these diseases by wearing gloves for longer hours in the cold.

Tips to Cleanse and Sanitize Products after Diaster

After a disaster, it is important to clean the surface to prevent the spread of illness and disease:

- Use soap and warm water to wash surfaces and follow the safety instructions written on the product. You can use household bleach to clean the surface and below safety guidelines will help you:
- There is no need to mix bleach with the other cleaner and ammonia
- Use gloves, boots and eye protectors of rubber and non-porous material
- Avoid breathing in the fumes of the product and let the fresh air in by opening the doors and windows

Tips to Rescue the Victim of Fire

- The fire can cause destruction in the blink of an eye, and it can quickly spread through the area. The fire victim requires your personal help and care; therefore, get in touch with a fire victim. It will help you to heal the wounds with some emotional support.

- Treat the wounds of fire victim and offer your personal care. Apply antiseptic creams on the wounds and offer your financial support to the victim.

- Offer clothes and food items because the fire can damage everything. You can become a volunteer to offer emotional and financial support to the fire victim.

- Check the pulse of the victim if he is breathing. You can give cardiopulmonary resuscitation to help him to regain the breathing.

- Check the burns and treat them according to their type because the most serious burns are required to be treated in the first place. Remove the clothes from the burns and use sterile pad moisture with cool water. If you don't have a sterile pad, then you can use a clean cloth or towel.

- The second-degree burns will be treated with the cool running water and wrap the wound loosely. You can give pain killer and ibuprofen to avoid pain and burning. The minor burns can also be treated in the same way of soothing under cool and running water.

Conclusion

A first aid kit contains all supplies in one location and you can easily access it to save an injured person. A good survival medicine kit will help you to save money and time. A ready-made first aid kit is available in the market, but it will be beneficial to prepare your own kit.

It will enable you to keep customized items in your first aid kit, such as medical suture, bandages, antiseptic, arm splints, pain medication, prescription medication, emergency tourniquet, burn salve, tweezers, etc.

There are some first aid treatments and techniques that you should learn to manage different wounds and health problems immediately. It is important to learn dressing, treatment for fever, burns, injuries and poisoning.

In an emergency situation, it is essential to learn different techniques to handle the situation. There are a few skills that you should learn to treat minor injuries and deep wounds to stop bleeding.

FREE BonusReminder

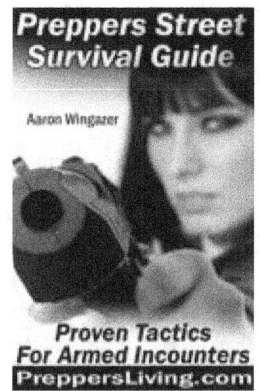

If you have not grabbed it yet, please go ahead and download your special bonus report *"DIY Projects. 13 Useful & Easy To Make DIY Projects To Save Money & Improve Your Home!"*

SimplyClicktheButtonBelow

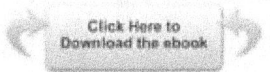

OR **Go to This Page**

http://preppersliving.com/free

BONUS #2: More Free & Discounted Books

Do you want to receive more Free & Discounted Books?

We have a mailing list where we send out our new Books when they go free or with a discount on Kindle. Click on the link below to sign up for Free & Discount Book Promotions.

=> Sign Up for Free & Discount Book Promotions <=

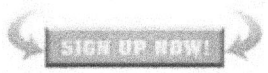

OR Go to this URL

http://zbit.ly/1WBb1Ek

www.ingramcontent.com/pod-product-compliance
Lightning Source LLC
Chambersburg PA
CBHW030104230526
45471CB00003B/1241